's

Perfect Postpartum Planning Worksheets

Table of Content

Congratulations! You're pregnant! This is such an exciting time in your life and nothing will ever truly be the same - for the better!

While pregnant with my oldest, I started planning my postpartum recovery. I wanted to have everything figured out so that the first weeks could run on autopilot. In retrospect, it was truly the best gift I could've given myself.

After giving birth, the body requires a *lot* of TLC before it is ready to start doing things again. We are constantly inundated with the idea that mom can bounce right back post-birth, but that is hardly the case:

Our organs need to move back into place and recover from the stress of pregnancy and childbirth.
Our bodies are rapidly going through hormonal and physiological changes.
Our brains are struggling to keep up with this new reality of life with a newborn while simultaneously adapting to the chemical changes.

Using these worksheets, I invite you to carve out a space to rest and focus on recovering after delivery. Resist the urge to go right back to "normal" life and give your body the time it needs to fully heal.

In health,

Hannah

How to Use the Worksheets

These worksheets will guide you through every aspect of your postpartum recovery.

i recommend working through these worksheets completely before beginning to purchase items, as you will be encouraged to sort items in a specific manner at the end of the worksheets.

A few of the worksheets are designed to be set out for visitors and family to reference. This includes freezer, fridge, and pantry lists, household task charts, and a to-do list at the end.

Describe your ideal postpartum recovery.

*My ideal postpartum recovery could be summed up like this:
The ability and freedom to exclusively rest/focus on the new baby and breastfeeding for the first 3-6 weeks. Once the bleeding slows down and no longer increases with activity, I will begin doing light walking and gentle pilates. Also, I will start to gradually handle the housework. I really want to tune into my body and how I am feeling on a day-to-day basis.*

Spotlight: Lying-In

What is Lying-In?

Lying-In is a period of time dedicated to allowing mom and baby rest following delivery. A mother's only job during this time is to breastfeed, eat, and rest.

Why the emphasis on Lying-In?

Traditionally, people viewed pregnancy and childbirth as extremely demanding for a mother - physically, mentally, and emotionally. The postpartum period was considered a crucial time for long term health and wellbeing. A woman's mother or female relatives were typically tasked with caring for the new mother and child during a set period of time.

Is Lying-In still relevent?

Absolutely! Women's bodies require six weeks for internal organ healing. There is some suggestion that women who observe a period of lying-in are less likely to experience postpartum mental health issues and improved breastfeeding. New mothers are often expected to bounce right back, which only feeds into mental health issues that plague moms today. Lying-In puts the housework and hosting on willing relatives/friends, giving mom the rest she needs.

Traditional approaches to Lying-In:

- Colonial America: 3-4 Weeks
- China: 30 Days
- Korea: 100 Days
- Malaysia: 30-44 Days
- India: 40-60 Days
- Jamaica: 8 Days
- Mexico: 40 Days
- Dominican Republic: 40 Days

From ravishly.com

Modern approaches to Lying-In:

- 10 Days of Lying-In
- 5 Days of Laying, 5 Days of Sitting, 5 Days of Seated Rest Allowing Guests
- 2 Weeks of Lying In + 4 Weeks of Limited Activity

Following delivery, how long do you wish to restrict all unnecessary movement and activity?

I recommend at least ten days of intentional rest following delivery to facilitate muscle recovery and trauma healing (i.e bruising) and encourage breastfeeding success.

    a. 30-40 Days (Traditional Recover Period - Long)
    b. 14-21 Days (Traditional Recovery Period - Short)
    c. 5 Days Laying, 5 Days Sitting (Modern Approach - More Rigid)
    d. 10 Days (Modern Approach - Moderate)
    e. Other:

How long do you wish to limit activity and movement?

I recommend avoiding all strenuous activity and exercise for six weeks following delivery to facilitate internal organ and pelvic floor healing.

    a. 12 Weeks
    b. 6 Weeks
    c. 3 Weeks
    d. Other:

Notes

What do you want other people to know about your postpartum recovery wishes?

The things I wanted everyone to know before delivery:
I want everyone to be on the same page about the importance and purpose of resting. I will sit down with key support people prior to delivery to share what has been prepared and what will need accomplished during my rest period. I also want to ask for no visitors the first 12-24 hours following delivery. We would like to take the time to rest and bond with our new baby.

6 Tips to Make Meal Prep Easier

#1 Emphasize shelf-stable items in the 1st & 2nd Trimesters

Homemade frozen meals tend to have a short-ish shelflife. Improper storage and freezer burn can impact the integrity of a meal. So, purchase all the shelf stable items (including toiletries and postpartum need) first and save frozen meals for the third trimester.

#2 Identify 3-5 meals your family loves that freeze well.

Don't try to plan a different meal each day. Make big batches of a select number of tried-and-true meals that you can count on. Be sure to freeze 1-3 Breakfast options in addition to the mains.

#3 Shoot for one big batch a week in the 3rd Trimester.

In order to make the most of your time and budget, aim for one big batch meal per week starting at 28 weeks and continue through week 35. Plan to freeze enough for 2 meals with every batch.

#4 Consider asking for food gift cards in your registry.

Inevitably, the first week of new parenthood is exhausting and other days pop up where the last thing you want to do is reheat a meal. Consider asking for food gift cards as an easy alternative to the meals you prepared.

#5 Don't count a meal train toward your total meal count.

When planning your meals, don't include an estimate of meals from a meal train. While it is very possible that you will be set for a few weeks following birth, it is also nice to have an additional stash set in place to take you that much further. If you are not anticipating a meal train, then be extra diligent to prepare a plethora of meals.

#6 Host a meal making party.

Not into slow and steady? Consider knocking it out in a day by calling in backup. This makes for a fun reason to get together with your friends!

Basic Calculations

Perfect Postpartum Planning Calculator

_______ x 7 = [ ]
(Weeks)   (Meal #)

How much do you need?

[ ] Breakfasts

[ ] Lunches

[ ] Dinners

How many weeks should you plan for?

Think through how long you'd like to be intentionally restful. (Refer back to previous worksheets for help with this.) We recommend preparing meals for at least that length of time *plus* two additional weeks. This gives you plenty of flexibility as you navigate your new routine.

Snack For Days Calculator

_______ x 3 = [ ]
(Meal #)   (Snack #)

How much do you need?

[ ] Snacks

Smart Snacking

Plan for more snacks than you think are necessary. Focus on a combination of options that are low in sugar while providing a balance of protein, fats, and carbs. Great options include protein bars, bananas with unsweetened yogurt and nuts, Ants on A Log, oatmeal bars, and trail mix.

Toiletry Calculator

How many toiletries do you go through in a month?

How much do you need?

_________ x 2 = [ ]
(Toilet Paper Use)

_________ x 2 = [ ]
(Paper Towel Use)

_________ x 2 = [ ]
(Laundry Detergent Use)

[ ] Toilet Paper

[ ] Paper Towels

[ ] Laundry Detergent

[ ]

[ ]

[ ]

Think through your basic toiletry needs for the month and plan to have twice as many purchased by the time you enter the third trimester. Add additional household items that you use on a regular basis.

Notes

Meal Brainstorming

<table>
<tr><td>

Breakfast

</td><td>

Lunch

</td></tr>
<tr><td>

Dinner

</td><td>

Snacks

</td></tr>
</table>

Emphasis: Nutrient Density

Pregnancy takes a lot out of a mom. One Australian Doctor has found a strong link between nutrient depletion in moms and mental health issues. I recommend creating your meal plan in a way that emphasizes nutrient dense foods over empty carbs and sugars to support a complete recovery.

Flexible Meal Plan

Breakfast	
Lunch	
Dinner	
Snacks	
Drinks	

Prefer a meal planning approach that is less rigid? Use this sheet to plan out a series of meals that suits your unique needs. Feel free to make multiple copies, if needed.

Structured Meal Plan

	Drinks	Snacks	Dinner	Lunch	Breakfast
Sunday					
Monday					
Tuesday					
Wednesday					
Thursday					
Friday					
Saturday					

Prefer having meals planned for specific days so you know that you've prepared enough?
Use this meal plan to meticulously plan the menu. Feel free to use multiple copies.

Freezer List

Meals	Sides	Misc.

Utilize this list to record what you have in the freezer.

Refrigerator List

Meals	Sides	Misc.

Utilize this list to record what you have in the pantry.

Pantry List

Snacks & Prepared	Ingredients	Misc.

Utilize this list to record what you have in the pantry.

Toiletries List

Bathroom	Pantry	Storage

Utilize this list to record your toiletries and their location..

Household Tasks

Bathrooms	
Laundry	
Kitchen	
Living Spacce	
Other	

Outline any recurring tasks that need done around the house.

Spotlight: Belly Band

What is belly binding?

Belly binding is the practice of wearing a girdle or belly bind postpartum to support internal healing.

What is the history of belly binding?

Belly wrapping is an old practice in Malaysian culture where it is known as "bengkung," and it has also been in practice in places like Japan and Mexico for hundreds of years. Women would wrap a piece of muslin or similar cloth around the abdomen of a new mom immediately after she had given birth to help give her extra physical support as her body healed.

History from care.com

How does belly binding support postpartum recovery?

- Encourages uterus to shrink back to original size.
- Gently supports the inner organs as they move back into place.
- Provides core support, allowing weakened muscles to recover.
- May encourage loose skin to tighten.

Types of Binds:

- Bengkung (Traditional Malaysian Bind)
- Girdle
- Girdle with Pants/Shorts (Similar to Shapewear)
- High Waisted Underwear/Girdle Hybrid
- Wrap
- Abdomen & Hip Band

Best for Small Budgets: 3-in-1 Postpartum Support (Amazon) or Women's High-Waisted Shapewear (Walmart)
Most Popular: Bellefit or Belly Bandit
My Personal Preference: Bengkung + Adjustable Wrap (Alternating Wear)

Looking for something?

Item	Find it here...

Offer instructions for finding certain items. i.e. Cleaning Supplies, Child's Clothing, Pizza Cutter, etc. Feel free to make extra copies.

Postpartum Recovery Needs

Clothing

i.e. Nursing Tanks, Underwear, etc.

Support Items

i.e. Belly Band, Frozen Pads, etc.

Supplements

i.e. DHA/DHEA, Vitamin D,
B-Complex, Mineral-Compex, etc.

Comfort

i.e. Essential Oils, Herb Bath Mix, etc.

Not sure what you will need for your postpartum recovery? Ask moms you know what they found to be the most useful items or look online for suggestions.

Postpartum Recovery Needs

Feminine Products

i.e. Heavy Pads, Wet Wipes, etc.

Support Items

i.e. Peri Bottle, Iodine, etc.

Natural Healing

i.e. Calendula Cream, EO Spray, etc.

Comfort

i.e. Extra Soft Toilet Paper, etc.

Not sure what you will need for your postpartum recovery? Ask moms you know what they found to be the most useful items or look online for suggestions.

What are your feeding plans?

Bottle Feeding i.e. breastpump, bottles, cooler, etc.

Breastfeeding i.e. Breast Pads, Boppy Pillow, Nipple Cream, etc.

Make a list of everything you need for diapering.

I encourage you to include extra clothing and burp clothes.

Where will you be spending most of your time?

a. Bedroom
b. Living Room
c. Family Room
d. Kitchen
e. Other:

How many bins do you need to assemble?

I encourage you to put together at least two bins. One for where you will spend time recovering postpartum and one for where you plan to sleep.

Snack & Activity Bins

Food

i.e. Bananas, Granola Bars, etc.

Drink

i.e. Water, Electrolyte Drink, etc.

Activities

i.e. Book, Remote, etc.

Practical

i.e. Phone Charger, Wipes, etc.

Put together a bin that you can keep near your dedicated spot for the first few weeks following delivery. If the bin is transportable, consider moving it to the bedroom at night.

Spotlight: Older Children

It is hard on older children to welcome a new sibling.

Inevitably, the attention shifts from the older children to the new baby and it can be hard on a family to make that transition. Regressions and trantrums are common and some experts theorize that these are an attempt to take back some of the previously given attention that is now missing.

What are some things you can do to make the transition a little bit easier?

- Talk about the new baby throughout the pregnancy.
- Talk about the things the new baby and your child can do together when he/she gets older.
- Incorporate the child as much as possible into the prep. Invite older children to help pick out something special for the baby to wear or organize items some of the caddies you have pre-planned.
- Set aside at least 10 minutes each day for 1-on-1 time with you and your significant other after the new baby is born.
- Use language and phrasing that reaffirms the child's place as a helper.
- Put together activity bins and special prizes for the child to to play with after the baby is born.
- Plan activities (i.e. sleepovers, play dates, etc.) that your child can look forward to after the baby is born.
- Purchase a doll for your child to dress, feed, change diapers, etc. as a way to normalize what is going to happen when the baby is born.

Who can you call to watch your child(ren) after the new baby is born?

Can your child(ren) stay with someone after the new baby is born? If so, list who.

How can you make your child(ren) feel special while recovering and caring for a new baby?

How can you help your child(ren) feel connected to - rather than competing with - the new baby?

Older Children's Bins

Activities

Consider assembling multiple caddies to rotate throughout the week.

Snacks

Consider assembling a help-yourself snack shelf.

Surprises & Treats

i.e. New Toy, Ice Cream, etc.

Together Activities

ie. Read A Book, etc.

We recommend filling out a copy of this page for each of your children (excluding baby).

Shopping Checklist & Timelines

1st Trimester

Congratulations! You're expecting! I encourage you to spend this time planning for your postpartum. Of course, no need to rush! Just set a goal of having the worksheets completed by start of the second trimester.

2nd Trimester

It's time to get down to business. Start planning to purchase 1-3 shelf stable foods, toiletries, and recovery items per week. Plan to knock out all of these before the third trimester.

This is a great time to make your baby registry and prepare for your shower!

3rd Trimester

This trimester, focus on stockpiling refrigerated items and preparing all the meals on your list. Be sure to leave reheating details with each meal. You can simply write instructions on aluminum foil or tape a note to the top of the dish.

Hopefully you've already had your baby shower! Use this time to finish purchasing your baby needs. If you don't mind second hand, consignment stores, thrift stores in upper class neighborhoods, and Facebook marketplace can be a great place to find quality items for cheap.

Grocery List

Meat	Dairy & Eggs	Dry Goods

Notes

Grocery List

Produce	Frozen	Misc.

Notes

Postpartum List

Clothing	Personal Care	Misc.

Notes

Big List of Postpartum Prep Tips

- **Label cabinets** - I used painter's tape and a marker to indicate what was in each. My husband thanked me a few weeks later.
- **Buy paper products** - Stock your cupboard with paper plates, disposable silverware, paper cups, and napkins to minimize the number of dishes that need washed in the first few weeks following delivery.
- **Do a pre-birth walkthrough** - Invite a family member or friend (or multiple) over to walk through the house before your give birth so you can verbally pass along instructions and answer questions.
- **Buy extra water bottles** - You need to be drinking a lot of water. Keep multiple, filled water bottles nearby to limit the number of refills you need during the day.
- **Put a list on the fridge** - Indicate what is available to be prepared and any tasks that need done. (There are pages included in this packet for you to utilize in preparing this list.)
- **Put a cooler on the front porch for food drop offs** - Don't feel obligated to invite everyone in. Communicate in advance that you would like to rest and will provide an opportunity to meet the baby at a later date.
- **Invest in a tablet** - Holding books and a newborn or breastfeeding isn't always realistic. Consider downloading ebooks, shows, etc. on a tablet to make the time go by faster.
- **Be proactive and ask people for help** - Other moms have been through this. Don't feel embarrassed to ask for help. If you don't have anyone nearby, consider asking a family member or friend to stay with you for a week (or more) following delivery.
- **Get your spouse on the same page** - Recovering from pregnancy and childbirth is hard. Educate your main support person on your postpartum wishes to minimize any struggles after baby is born.
- **Order extra vitamins** - Pregnancy leaves women in a depleted state that is linked to postpartum mental health issues, breastfeeding struggles, stubborn weight, and more. Continue taking your prenatal after delivery and consider adding in DHA/DHEA, Vitamin D, and a mineral supplement, in addition to a nutrient-dense meal plan.

Second Trimester Shopping List

Emphasis: Household Items
& Recovery Needs

Use this page to separate the shopping list by trimester.

Third Trimester Shopping List

Emphasis: Food

Use this page to separate the shopping list by trimester.

Thanks for stopping by! Here are a few things you can do to support us before you leave.